HEALTHY LIVING

Mental Health, Find Happiness by Improving Your Gut Health, Sugar Addiction & IBS

Maria Lexington

Maria Lexington

Table of Contents

INTRODUCTION...7

CHAPTER 1: GETTING STARTED 9

CHAPTER 2: SIBO.. 13

CHAPTER 3: IRRITABLE BOWEL SYNDROME 21

CHAPTER 4: WHAT IS DOPAMINE? 29

CHAPTER 5: SUGAR ADDICTION & THE GUT.....................33

CHAPTER 6: MEDICATIONS & SUPPLEMENTS 43

CHAPTER 7: HERBAL TREATMENT 47

CHAPTER 8: SPECIFIC CARBOHYDRATE DIET 53

CHAPTER 9: PALEO DIET 61

CHAPTER 10: GAPS DIET 69

CHAPTER 11: FODMAP DIET...81

CHAPTER 12: REPLACEMENTS 85

CONCLUSION 95

Maria Lexington

Introduction

I want to thank you and congratulate you for purchasing the book, *"SIBO Cure: How to Overcome SIBO and Heal Your Gut"*.

This book contains proven steps and strategies on how to use Medicinal, Natural remedies, Diet, and Lifestyle changes to heal small intestinal bacteria overgrowth and restore your gut health.

The book is all about Small Intestinal Bacterial Overgrowth, starting from its background and going right into its treatment. In the middle however, it tells you about the potential causes, symptoms and complications of the condition so you would be at a higher ground right from the beginning.

As you read on you will find out that the disease is much serious than you thought but don't worry as all the cures you need have been provided in the book: artificial or natural, you name it. I've given medicinal cures firstly so your take-the-pill instinct would be satisfied.

Next, I've given the natural herbs treatment for SIBO followed by Dietary treatment, spearheaded by the Specific Carbohydrate Diet which I found to be the most effective against SIBO. Step-by-step instruction has been provided wherever necessary; the information in the book is complete, well-researched and managed so you will have the best chances to fight off the condition, for once and for all.

Thanks again for purchasing this book, I hope you enjoy it!

Chapter 1

Getting Started

Bacteria play an essential role in maintaining a healthy gut & perform important functions that help in proper digestion but sometimes their overgrowth in the small intestinal tract can lead to more problems than solutions.

The small intestine that connects the stomach with the large intestine is almost 20 feet in length with bacteria being present throughout the tract, but in different concentrations at different places. Few bacteria inhibit the small intestine compared to the large one or even the colon where at least 1,000,000,000 bacteria/milliliter are present. Moreover, the types of bacteria in different parts of the gut are not all the same.

The small intestinal is vital for the process of digestion & absorption of nutrients and contains a sophisticated network of lymphoid cells, which are integral for top-notch immunity. As stated earlier, the normal bacteria play an essential part in the small bowel by fighting off pathogens and yeast; they also help in the absorption of nutrients like vitamins, fatty acids, folic acid, etc. It is due to these bacteria that food moves in the small intestine with relative ease. When the type or number of bacteria in the small intestine change, it is then that a person is at risk of developing the condition known as small intestinal bacterial overgrowth. But before you can move on to that, you must know the importance of the small intestine in the gut.

The gut, as many of you might know is a long tube that stretches from the mouth to the anus. The first part of the gut is the mouth from where food is consumed; the food then passes down into the stomach through the esophagus and from there it enters the small intestine. The small intestine has three parts namely:

    i.   Duodenum,

    ii.   Jejunum,

    iii.   Ileum,

The first part follows on from the stomach and curls around the pancreas forming a C shape. The second & third part makes up the rest of the intestine and is coiled in the abdomen. In here, the nutrients are absorbed from where it is passed onto the large intestine. The large intestine continues upwards until it joins the colon, which ultimately leads to the rectum from where waste materials are passed on.

The gut is responsible for processing food, right from the time it enters our mouth and until it is passed out through the anus. Each part of the gut plays some role in the whole digestive system and one cannot be given precedence over the other. Therefore, even if a single organ in the gut malfunctions, the whole body suffers as a result. Some disorders that can be caused due to problems in the gut include:

- Acid reflux,

- Appendicitis,

- Cystic fibrosis,

- Small Intestinal Bacterial Overgrowth,

- Diarrhea,

- Stomach cancer,

- Hernia,

- Gallstones,

- Threadworms,

- Ulcers,

Small intestine is a part of the gut and therefore, SIBO as well is a condition that affects the whole gut. As you read on, you will find out that SIBO has connections with many other ailments in the gut, therefore, making its cure essential for the proper health of the body.

Maria Lexington

Chapter 2

SIBO

Undoubtedly bacteria are essential for the process of digestion in the body but most bacteria in the gastrointestinal tract should be present in the large intestine & colon instead of the small intestine. When this does not happen, the body starts suffering from various conditions that can be attributed to Small Intestinal Bacterial Overgrowth.

Most people suffer from SIBO, not due to the overgrowth of a single type of bacteria but due to various types of bacteria working in conjunction. Once you suffer from SIBO, both the function & the structure of your small intestine and thus the gut will take a toll. There will be severe interference in the process of digestion & absorption of nutrients due to damaged cell linings. This damage may even cause leaky gut which is an inflammatory disease that makes the intestinal barrier more permeable, resulting in undigested particles getting absorbed! This disease itself has several negative effects that include immune complications, food allergies & generalized inflammation.

On top of the poor absorption function that is already present, the bacteria can cause nutritional deficiencies, meaning that it will absorb some vitamins & minerals before they get absorbed. Some instances of protein deficiency have also been recorded whereby the bacteria absorb amino acids. Methane & hydrogen gas are also a byproduct of early breakdown of nutrients by the bacteria that can cause bloating, flatulence, belching, cramping, IBS and even diarrhea. The gas trouble does not stop here, and this pressure can make the gas travel upwards leading to the development of hiatal hernia, heartburn, nausea and acid reflux.

Causes of SIBO:

Medical practitioners believe that some conditions can aid in the growth of excess bacteria that upsets the normal balance of things. These include:

- Decreased motility – this condition is caused due to excess dietary sugar, diabetes, scleroderma, hypothyroidism and chronic stress.

- Hypochlorhydria – with the passage of time, the amount of acid released in the stomach decreases with makes the gut more prone to bacterial overgrowth. One of the acids that lead to the inhibition of SIBO is hydrochloric acid or HCL, which not only helps in the digestion of proteins but also prevents bacteria from forming colonies. If there is a shortness of this acid in the body then SIBO is imminent.

- Structural abnormalities – blind loop, gastric bypass surgery, small intestinal diverticula, Crohn's disease; these are some of the abnormalities that lead to SIBO.

- Stress – this can play a huge role in low levels of hydrochloric acid as well as intestinal motility due to the inhibition of digestive secretion by the nervous system. When a person is relaxed the nervous system is also at its peak and the overall rate of digestion is improved but too much worries can disrupt the functions of small intestine placed to defend against bacterial overgrowth, leading to SIBO.

- Faulty ileocecal valve – this normally closed duct separates the small & large intestines, required to prevent flow of materials from the large intestine to the small one. When there is a malfunction in this valve, materials including bacteria can travel up the intestine causing several conditions, one of which is SIBO.

- Other causes may include stress, antibiotics, steroids, birth control mechanisms & enzyme deficiency.

Symptoms of SIBO:

A precise estimate of the number of people suffering from this condition is still unknown but studies have suggested that 6 – 15% of the general population suffers from this condition; it was also found that 80% of IBS patients have this syndrome. Bacterial overgrowth is a condition that may be present in the small intestine for years before a formal symptom surfaces. It is due to this reason that SIBO is left undiagnosed. But when symptoms worsen, a trip to the doctor is necessary where many tests are taken to determine the condition. You can self-diagnose the condition yourself as the symptoms are quite easy to read (and feel!):

- Abdominal discomfort,

- Diarrhea,

- Bloating,

- Constipation,

- Gas & belching,

- Leaky gut,

- Auto-immune disorders,

- Pain in multiple joints,

- Sever cases even cause weight loss,

Now, you may have a question about the spread of SIBO, i.e. "Is SIBO contagious?" The answer is No. Unlike many bacterial conditions in the gut, SIBO is not contagious. Studies have shown that a single microorganism is not responsible for the outbreak of SIBO, but a multitude of bacteria cause it.

Risk Factors of SIBO:

There are several risk factors that come with having the Small intestinal bacterial overgrowth. There are mainly three types of risk factors that people are exposed to, they are: one, immunity disorders where in your immune system and metabolism is affected, two, risk factors that include more bacteria growth or the movement of bacteria from colon to the small bowel and difficulty in the movement of the small bowel. There can also be anatomical changes that can cause issues like the restriction of movement of fluids and liquids. Other problems that can arise due to SIBO include motility problems where the free movement of bowel may get restricted and get diffused.

Other risk factors include ailments like scleroderma, which is an autoimmune disease, which hardens skin and internal organs causing slow bowel movements. This slow bowel movement is attributed towards increase in the concentration of bacteria. Celiac disease is another autoimmune disease that is based on the small intestine causing pain, diarrhea and so on. This disease too can contribute to the increase in the amount of bacteria present in the small intestine. Out pouchings are commonly called diverticulas wherein a hollow organ or an organ that contains fluids starts to pouch. This can occur in the small bowel causing the accumulation of bacteria. The Blind loop syndrome, which occurs from surgery of the stomach and duodenum, can also cause the slow movement of fluids in the bowel.

Other intestinal liquids and juices also become slow in their movement causing a bacterial overgrowth over a period of time. There are several risk factors that are yet to be considered, these include immune system disorders like pancreatitis. Pancreatitis is called the inflammation of the pancreas and this inflammation can cause several bacteria to infest and multiply leading to bacterial overgrowth. Even medication can put one under risk when coming to SIBO. In fact, several researches show that immunosuppressant medications are those that can easily cause an overgrowth of bacteria. Genetic deficiencies especially those like immunodeficiency conditions like that of IgA deficiency, combined variable immunodeficiency and hypogammaglobulinemia can also put one under the risk of developing an overgrowth of bacteria in their small intestines.

Apart from just these, any problems that occur between the channels of the colon and the small bowel can cause issues, this is because the colon is infested with several bacteria and any passage that is faulty can make the bacteria shift to the small bowel increasing the bacterial content in the small bowel. This is especially true with people who have Crohn's disease. Others who have problems with ileocecal valve can also develop an overgrowth of bacteria. This is because the ileocecal valve connects both the small bowel and large bowel and any problems in this can increase the amount of bacteria in the small bowel. This is specific to people who have the ileocecal valve removed from their systems through surgery like those of bariatric surgery.

Other people who are at risk include those who utilize the proton pump inhibitors to reduce the amount of acid in the stomach. This can increase the risk of acquiring SIBO. Currently there are several research and experiments that are being undertaken by scientists and doctors to establish the connections between the risk factors associated with SIBO.

Others who happen to have the irritable bowel syndrome can be at a higher risk of developing an increase in the influx of bacteria in their small intestine. In fact, recent studies and research has shown that about 75 to 80 per cent of the people who have irritable bowel syndrome develop an increase in the amount of bacteria in their system. This is especially true in the cases of those who underwent the hydrogen breath test. However this test also has been criticized for showing false positives in many cases. This is because the fermentation methodology and the timing of the breath test generally give a positive result for SIBO. But further studies have shown that those who have taken treatment for SIBO have felt a reduction in their irritable bowel syndrome.

Those who have fibromyalgia also are at a risk of developing bacteria accumulation in their small intestines. Breath tests have shown that those with condition have more bacteria in their small intestines. There are also several researches that have shown that there is a positive link between those with fibromyalgia and SIBO. This is because though fibromyalgia is a condition that is associated with pain, it results in the development of high levels of intestinal hyperpermeability, which can cause SIBO. Rosacea is a chronic skin condition and those with this condition are at a higher risk of developing an increase in the amount of bacteria in their small intestine.

Recent studies and research have concluded that people with rosacea have been tested using the hydrogen breath test to detect SIBO and that those with rosacea have their test results come out positive. This implies an increase in the presence of bacteria. These patients whose test results came out positive were given antibiotics like rifaximin for a period of one week to ten days. These antibiotics were non absorbable in nature and did not leave the digestive tract. When this was done, those with rosacea received a remission of their symptoms and discomforts. Those patients whose tests came out negative were also retested only to find that there was bacterial overgrowth. There were also some cases of relapse of rosacea in some patients, which got cleared, with additional doses of non-absorbable antibiotics. Alternate studies have used methane breath tests for rosacea patients instead of hydrogen based breath test. This has proved to be futile with the injection of antibiotics like rifaximin. However, they were also given alternate antibiotics, which targeted intestinal bacteria, which in turn reduced their symptoms of rosacea.

There are also suggestions made by doctors and scientists, which state that the type of antibiotic varies depending on the person's constitution. However studies have shown that with the correct usage of antibiotics, which target the intestinal bacteria, the symptoms of rosacea have come down.

Treatment:

This book will guide you through 3 ways, which you may utilize for curing SIBO. I will leave no stone unturned and provide the information in the most comprehensive manner possible so you get rid of the irritating disease, in the shortest span of time. The book treats SIBO through:

i.   Medications, both antibiotics and supplements,

ii.   Natural cures which include herbs,

iii.   Diets, which include Low FODMAPs and Paleo Diet.

Read on and find out more.

Chapter 3
Irritable Bowel Syndrome

While there are many gastrointestinal diseases that can plague the stomach like Celiac disease, Crohn's disease, etc., IBS or irritable bowel syndrome is the one that truly stands out for its effects on the body in general which are very much linked to addiction to sugar. But what exactly is IBS?

Irritable bowel syndrome is a disorder in the gut that is functional in nature meaning that nothing is wrong with the structure of the gut but the functionality isn't as expected. Thus, in irritable bowel syndrome only the function of the gut is upset and otherwise the gut looks quite normal, e.g. when looked under the microscope. Almost 1 in every 5 individual in the UK is known to suffer from IBS during some part of his/her life and even though IBS is known to strike at any age, it usually affects youngsters and women.

Symptoms:

There are a number of symptoms of IBS that a person has to suffer through. These are:

1. Pain & discomfort – this may occur in various parts of the abdomen. The pain usually fades in and fades out whereas the interval is unexpected as well as the time when it can strike. The pain goes away or becomes less intensified when you pass a stool. Many people who suffer from IBS describe the pain as something of a spasm over which they have no control. In addition, the severity of the pain can also vary from one person to the other as well as from one episode to the next, so this is really not something you should put up with and should look for a cure right away, as given in the book.

2. Bloating – the abdomen may swell and feelings of bloating may fade in from time to time.

3. Stooling pattern – People may suffer from episodes of diarrhea while others may suffer from constipation. Some people even suffer from both of these conditions alternatively. Many times the stools can be watery and may have mucus with them.

   Furthermore, people who suffer from IBS always have a feeling of not emptying up after having been to the toilet. There can also be urgency to go to the bathroom at various moments that can disrupt day-to-day routine life.

4. Other symptoms:

   - Nausea,

   - Belching,

   - Headache

- Muscle pain,

- Tiredness,

- Heartburn,

- Poor appetite,

- Cravings for a particular food

Causes:

The symptoms may very well be distinct but the causes are still ambiguous. However, common ground has been found and one or more of the following may be the reason as to why you are suffering from the gut-wrenching disease.

- IBS may be caused by over activity of the nerves located in the gut. The reason as to why this might happen isn't quite known but it has been found that too much communication between the gut and the brain can cause this condition. In addition, stress & emotional factors also play a huge role. Almost half of the people who suffer from IBS have related their happening to a stressful event in their life. It has also been found that symptoms get worse as a person goes through stressful events.

- Intolerance to a specific good group may also play its part and cause IBS but this cause hasn't been proven yet.

- Infections or too much bad bacteria in the gut can also trigger Irritable Bowel Syndrome. In many cases the symptoms soon appear after a person suffers from a consecutive cycle of diarrhea, vomiting and constipation.

- Oversensitivity to pain may also be a cause to IBS as people may feel discomfort as their gut expands.

Risk Factors for Those with IBS:

Studies have shown that those with irritable bowel syndrome happen to develop malfunctioning in their gut. The flora of the bacteria present over there decreases and this is more prominent with those suffering from diarrhea predominant IBS. Thus there is a development of antibodies like flagellin in the gut that will affect the bacteria present in it. These antibodies also cause mild inflammation of the gut along with other changes and malfunctions like intraepithelial lymphocytes, increased enterochromaffin cells and mast cells. Alternately there are several other factors that can cause the risk of acquiring IBS these includes both genetic factors and environmental factors. In terms of genetics, people who hail from families with multiple cases of IBS usually report symptoms and signs of IBS.

Other factors that can cause the development of IBS include consumption of certain foods like extremely spicy foods. IBS affects women more than men and the lifestyle choices play a crucial role in this. Other factors like changes in the serotonin metabolisms can also result in the development of IBS. In fact, studies show that people who have a high level of serotonin transporter in the ileum are those who are suffering from IBS. Other studies have also confirmed that an increase in the number of apoptotic genes in the irritable bowel syndrome can account to the development of a large quantity of mast cells in the intestine, which can cause problems including internalization of protein components of the gut like occludin and ZO-1.

Most commonly genetics play a crucial role in determining who acquires IBS. Therefore any genetic problems and defects are directly linked to the severity of IBS. Defects in the epithelial homeostasis and the innate immunity can induce the risk of developing several types of IBS including the post infectious variety. There is also evidence that claims that those with severe forms of gastroenteritis infection can develop symptoms of IBS. Usually, the genetic factors don't get triggered unless there is some severe malfunction like that in the epithelial barriers however they can be contributed by high levels of stress and anxiety, which can cause post infectious forms of IBS. One of the major characteristics of the post infectious IBS is that it is a type of diarrhea predominant IBS. This has been found through tests that have shown a large quantity of emissions of proinflammatory cytokines. This happens due to enteric infection. This in turn can cause perforations in the gut causing gut permeability. When this takes place, the bacteria found can get transported due to the breaking of the epithelial barriers through the gut perforations causing severe damage to the linings and tissues. This will lead to further complexities especially to those who are sensitive to gut problems. Regardless of the type of infection that can trigger IBS, any increase in the gut permeability has always been linked to IBS.

Scientists and doctors are constantly researching on the IBS and in the 1990s several publications and research thesis came about showing psychological links to IBS. In fact, studies claim that any physical abuse, mental torment and psychological issues like blackmail and insecurity can cause IBS triggers. This is probably because anxiety and stress play a crucial role in developing IBS and when psychological and physical issues stem in, it can create complications. It can also lead to several other symptoms like fibromyalgia and chronic fatigue syndrome, which can increase the stress levels and cause acute IBS. The studies that were conducted in the 1990s show that the stress hormone in the brain involves the nervous systems along with HPA axis and these malfunction in the cases of those with irritable bowel syndrome. Therefore any psychiatric illness pertaining to anxiety can result in the development of IBS. In fact, studies show that 2 out of 3 people with stress level illness develop high levels of irritable bowel syndrome.

Other studies also show links between those with small intestinal bacterial overgrowth and those with IBS. In fact, IBS occurs most commonly in those who suffer from an influx of bacteria in their gut. Most often, the patients diagnosed with SIBO develop symptoms of diarrhea predominant IBS. There are also several cases where constipation predominant IBS can also be triggered through SIBO. They also develop into symptoms like diarrhea or constipation, bloating, abdominal pain, and other such signs. Other risk factors include those of faulty interactions between the bacteria in the gut and those in the immune systems. This can cause increase in the amount of cytokine signaling profile.

Further studies have also confirmed that any changes that occur in the gut especially in the levels of bacteria present in the gut can cause problems in the intestines. These problems in the intestines can cause IBS. This can also be triggered by psychiatric problems. 80 per cent of the people with problems in their gut develop the symptoms of IBS. Studies are being currently undertaken by scientists and doctors to find links between the sudden increase in the amount of yeast; especially in Candida Albicans in the flora of the gut and the symptoms of IBS. Other types of research include those where the scientists are trying to establish links between protozoal infections like that of blastocystosis and IBS. This is because people with IBS have also complained about having developed protozoal infections especially the organism Dientamoeba fragilis.

Food sensitivities can also trigger problems with respect to IBS. Studies have thrown light on the fact that consumption of wheat, dairy, and sugary fruits rich in fructose or sugary substitutes like sorbitol can trigger symptoms. Other foods like fatty foods; alcohol and fizzy drinks like soda and aerated drinks can also cause imbalance the bacterial flora found in the gut and upset the digestive system causing it. Eating large meals and eating after stressful activities like exercises can cause IBS. Antidepressant medications and those containing sorbitol and even food poisoning can increase the risk of developing IBS.

Treatments:

The treatments are very much similar to those used for Small Intestinal Bacterial Overgrowth that can be attained through a series of lifestyle changes. The Specific Carbohydrate Diet given later on will very much help you attain this goal so I strongly recommend you follow it in addition to a couple of dietary guidelines given below:

- Enjoy regular meals and don't be in a rush while eating; choose a time when you don't have to worry about other unfinished businesses.

- Avoid skipping meals or going without eating anything substantial, i.e. natural for days.

- Set your minimum fluid consumption to 8 cups/day especially drinks that aren't caffeinated. Water in particular will help normalize your bowel movements.

- Restricts caffeinated drinks to 3 cups/day; caffeine needs to be given special attention as it can be a frequent trigger to IBS. It goes for fizzy and carbonated drinks too.

- Avoid drinking too much alcohol, restricting yourself to the amount that gets you through the day.

- Limit intake of high-fiber food,

- Eat at least 3x, 80 grams portion of fresh fruit every day,

- If you suffer from episodes of diarrhea then avoid sorbitol, artificial sweetener that can be found in a variety of chewing gums, drinks and slimming products.

- Increase your intake of oats and linseeds if bloating does not go away from the Specific Carbohydrate Diet.

It can be seen that many of the symptoms coincide with the symptoms of Small Intestinal Bacterial Overgrowth given in the previous chapter that shows one essential thing: it's all linked to the gut.

The revelation may be unsurprising but the fact is that poor gut health can result in a number of problems, simultaneously or individually which can only be cured through serious changes in one's lifestyle. As you read on you will find out that gut isn't as isolated as you think it is and is in heavy contact with the brain. In fact it effects' the brain's decision, especially food-related ones and poor gut health can give way to unnecessary cravings, one of which is sugar addiction.

Chapter 4

What is Dopamine?

Before I move right into the specifics of Sugar Addiction and how Gut Health is related to it, you must be told about Dopamine, a chemical that is one of the root causes of Substance addiction and is very much linked to the gut.

Sugar isn't something man created, it isn't something artificial and it's been around since the advent on mankind. So why do we get addicted with the natural product sugar, instead of foods like oatmeal, cabbage, potato, etc. Point to ponder, isn't it. This point in particular has been the subject of scientific researches, i.e. why carbohydrate rich foods are addictive while others aren't, for decades now and researchers have figured it out to some extent, linking it to the receptor dopamine.

Think of dopamine as a receptor in our brain that is activated every time you feel pleasure or satiety. This neurotransmitter in particular is one of the biggest causes of most addictions as it has been found through research that sugars, i.e. carbohydrates and alcohol are its biggest activators. It has also been found that sugar holds greater power & influence than the illicit drug heroin when it comes to activating dopamine. The chemical structure of sugar and alcohol is quite similar which is one of the reasons they top the list but another reason as to why sugar cravings are so much connected to dopamine is due to the Gut-Brain connection, as you'll see later on.

Dopamine isn't entirely bad and controlled production is necessary to keep the body out of depression however when a person finds a particular substance, in this case, sugar, which helps him/her to forcefully activate this receptor, he/she starts abusing it. Production of excess dopamine can provide more satisfaction and pleasure but with the passage of time the body starts to develop resistance to sugar and soon overeating begins which leads to addiction. Furthermore, the brain becomes highly dependent on a particular substance like sugar to maintain normal dopamine levels and as soon as the reserves run out the person starts to feel down, depressed, and a host of other conditions like lack of focus, mood swings, and etc. until he/she is given another dose of sugar.

The entire process of sugar addiction is a deceptive ones and an individual never knows or admits he is addicted until the signs become unavoidable. With that being said, you must also understand that there isn't only a single aspect, i.e. dopamine that controls sugar addiction. Dopamine itself is linked to a number of aspects and other physical conditions as well are responsible for sugar addiction. Another hormone in particular that comes out fat cells also plays a huge role in "telling" dopamine that there is enough sugar in the body. The hormone sends a signal to the brain as soon as sugar enters the body but with the passage of time the hormones also develop resistance that means more & more sugary products are required to release it and send a signal to the brain.

Now that you know the role played by dopamine you'll be able to understand the link between gut bacteria as well as other ailments and cravings in general. The next chapter discusses the basics of sugar addiction followed by the problems in a person's digestive tract that support this problem.

Maria Lexington

Chapter 5

Sugar Addiction & the Gut

Everyone loves to consume sugary products, whether it's in the form of natural food items like fruits or artificial ones like muffins, brownies, a can of coke, etc. Unknowingly, we make sugary products a regular part of our diet and soon they become an essential rather than an expendable portion of our meal plan. Without a sugary treat, we feel confused, tired, annoyed, and physically ill but as soon as they body is fed with something sweet, the brain becomes stable and the whole body comes to peace. But as time passes, some people start to realize the roots of their addiction and when they try to let go of it, they fail miserably and have to start consumption once again due to the host of diseases withdrawal gives rise to. Sugar has a widespread effect on the body's natural settings, especially hormonal levels, as explained in the previous chapter so as soon as the person tries to quit it, he faces a plethora of other diseases.

There are a number of reasons as to why a person may become addicted to sugar; some are physical while some are psychological. A person may have been through a depressive event or a trauma and found sugar as his/her salvation. A person may have "casually" consumed sugar for so long that now he/she can't operate normally without it or a person may be suffering from one or many underlying conditions which would've forced him/her to resort to sugar.

The last of the reasons is the focus of this particular book.

The first physical cause of sugar addiction is an infection in the brain known as "brain-yeast infection". This nifty yet dangerous problem evolves with the development of yeast in the brain that feeds off sugar. The yeasts produces a small amount of alcohol as soon as it gets a little sugar which gives the body a little high, courtesy of dopamine! Naturally, when the yeast does not get the appropriate amount of sugar, the "high" disappears and the person goes through recurring episodes of anxiety, depression and anger. This is one of the zones where sugar addiction has been found linked to dopamine.

The next condition that has been identified as the cause of sugar addiction has its epicenter in the gut, i.e. hypoglycemia. It is well known that consumed sugar is converted into glucose so it can be used in the body. In normal condition, the body does not require excess amount of sugar, but instead requires a balanced diet. The balanced diet may include fats, proteins, carbohydrates, vitamins, etc. which are all broken down into bits of foods that can be digested. However, in case of a bad digestive system, the person starts craving simple sugars that are found in honey, fruit, junk foods, etc. These cravings only surface when the body isn't able to digest complex bits of foods, which means that the gut isn't working, as it was supposed to. The consumption of simple sugars that are harmful for the body soon turns into addiction giving birth to a plethora of other conditions.

Hypoglycemia can very well be analogized with a clogged fuel system of a car. Gasoline travels through a series of filtrations and processes before it reaches the engine but if any of these processes does not work, by passing these steps may make a car unstable or not work at all. It is the case for the human body where the gut acts as the passageway for food; an incomplete or impaired function within the gut would mean a non-functioning human body.

Now do you understand the importance of the gut and the role it plays in keeping addictions like sugar at bay? Read on and find out more as to how healing the gut would help the body get rid of its sugar addiction.

A Troubled Fuel System

Food must pass through various portions of the gut and must undergo the respective processes before reaching the liver where it is converted to glucose and moving onto the small intestine. A dysfunctional organ anywhere along this path can result in a chain-reaction and a problem for the whole system since there isn't any by-pass pipeline!

The basic processes that await the food as it enters the gut can be summarized as:

- Food items like carbohydrates, fats & proteins are consumed.

- Digestion begins in the mouth as the saliva starts breaking down food to make it easier for the gut to digest,

- As the semi-broken down foo reaches the stomach, the digestion process continues; hydrochloric acid in the stomach as well as other enzymes mix in with the food to break it down further.

- Next, the food enters the small intestine where it is mixed up with bile and pancreatic juices that further digest the food.

- The food is now broken down into its constituents, i.e. carbohydrates are converted to sugars, and fats are converted to fatty acids while proteins are converted to amino acids. These broken down bits are then absorbed into the lower intestine from where they move onto other organs like the kidney and liver.

- When they enter the liver, the bits are converted into nutrients that can essentially be used by the body. Sugars are converted to glycogen and get passed into the bloodstream whereas the kidneys are responsible for removing harmful products out of the digested food.

- Next, the nutrients exit the liver and get injected into the body's cells that mean that they must pass through cell membranes that are activated by the infamous hormone insulin.

- From there the nutrients enter the cell where they are converted into a chemical that can be harnessed by the cell's powerhouse known as adenosine triphosphate.

That was the overall view of what goes inside the body, mostly the gut when food is eaten. However, as mentioned, problems can arise which can lead to impaired digestion and thus sugar addiction.

One of these problems is known as "Candida Yeast Infection" that can plague that gastrointestinal tract, which is part of the gut. The gut consists of both good bacteria as well as bad bacteria. Candida, a yeast competes with the good bacteria for greater space within the gut; a healthy diet consisting of probiotic food items can keep the gut safe from any such infections however too little amount of good bacteria in the gut can lead to Candida overgrowth.

This Candida yeast feeds off sugar in the gastrointestinal tract and as soon as the sugar levels hit rock bottom, the yeast gives rise to sugar cravings. But giving the yeast more sugar will only increase its presence in the gut as it will regenerate and spread throughout the gut, which in turn will make you want to eat more sugar. The process will continue and before you know it you'll be a sugar addict. And because sugar is known to disrupt the body's natural immunity response, the body is helpless in front of this yeast that slowly takes over the intestinal wall leading to irritation both internally and externally.

The gut is sometimes called the "second brain" of the human body as it shares a number of properties & characteristics of the real one! The gut is made up of several types of neurons along with a blood-brain barrier that keeps its stable. In addition, the gut also releases a number of hormones and neurotransmitters (over 40), similar to those found in the brain. The neurons in the gut are also responsible for generating the infamous hormone dopamine as well as 95 percent of the hormone serotonin that circulates in the body.

As it has been previously told that in the brain, the hormone dopamine is responsible for making the person "feel good". It has a similar function in the gut where it coordinates between the various neurons that line the gut and the brain. On the other hand, production of serotonin also depends on the condition of gut so every time the gut feels stable or it "thinks" that it feel stable, the hormone is released that results in better body temperature, appetite and mood. The serotonin is in no way limited to the gut and spreads throughout the body after entering the bloodstream where it repairs the lungs & liver.

But how does the gut control our mood and cravings? There is no doubt about the fact that the gut doesn't have emotions, but nonetheless it does have an influence over them! Researchers have carried out a number of studies and have concluded that neurotransmitters released in the gut can't reach the brain however it has been found small gaps in the blood-brain barrier can allow such an event. But even if the neurotransmitters don't reach the brain, the gut can still influence the brain's emotion through nerve transmissions.

In fact, these are the very signals that are responsible for cravings and explain why sugary & fatty foods make us feel good about ourselves. When sugary foods are ingested, they are detected by receptors in the gut that in turn send signals to the brain to release feel-good neurotransmitters. Such a response does not come in normal conditions and is only generated when lining in the gut is not functioning properly, which may be due to a disease, condition or an ailment.

Therefore, the only way to get over such cravings and beat sugar addiction is to combat the problems that reign the gut including SIBO, IBS and other digestive-tract issues. All of these cannot be left for our immunity to cure as the chronic cycle of sugar addiction also throws the immune system out of balance, which means that the immune system isn't even able to detect issues with the gut. Thus, only drastic measures that cure the gut can ultimately help you get over your sugar addiction; otherwise, if you rule out gut abnormalities, then you'll only have a short-term cure and it'll be a matter of days, weeks or months before sugar addiction strikes again.

In this section of the book we look at the various ways through which you can reduce your sugar cravings. Discussed below are some tips and tricks to reduce your sugar cravings.

1. It is important to know that the more sugar you eat, the more sugar you will crave. So focus on cutting down sugar gradually and not eradicating it completely at once. For instance, if you take three sugar cubes in your coffee or tea, then you can cut down to having two sugar cubes and so on. Try this for a week or a few days and then later on you can cut down to one sugar cube. Similarly if you take two bars of chocolates, cut down to one. Take it slow. There are times when you can go cold turkey and remove all sugars from your diet for a few days. This however has very few success rates.

2. It is a good idea to combine foods. Instead of having one whole carton of sweet juice, mix it with some water. Dilute the amount of sugar to reduce the amount of sugar you are consuming. Opt for the ratio 1:1. If you are finding this hard, then you can add 3/4th glass of water and then gradually increase it. Similarly, instead of a bowl of sweetened yogurt you can take half a cowl of sweetened yogurt mixed with plain and fresh yogurt. You can also consume healthier options along with the sugary goods. For instance you can take some strawberry with chocolate. This way you also get some nutrients in.

3. There are several studies that have shown that people who suffer from acute sugar cravings have been able to reduce it by using gum. When you manage to get sugar cravings, pop some gum instead. The enzymes present in the gum are said to reduce your sugar cravings.

4. Opt for healthy sugar instead of the sugary junk that you usually crave. If you are craving for chocolates then it is a good idea to consume fruits that are sweet instead. Consume apples and bananas as these are sweet and can reduce the sweet cravings that you suffer from. These

fruits also contain huge amounts of fibers and other important nutrients that are abundantly healthier than sugary substances. They also have natural sugars in them, which are far healthier like fructose. You can also opt for dried fruits and sweet nuts.

5. Eat regularly and break your meals into small sizes. This can actually help you because sugar craving usually starts when you go hungry. If you take your meals regularly and break your meals into small bite size proportions you will be able to reduce your cravings. Irrational eating can lead to digestive problems and it gives you more time to go hungry. Also when you do not eat regularly you start opting for fatty sugary foods that can hinder your hunger. They fill you up and are unhealthy. Taking regular meals will ensure that you get adequate nutrients and you do not load up on junk. This can also prevent future problems from occurring.

6. Have a specific amount of sugar that you can consume per day. It might be shocking to know but an average person consumes close to 20 teaspoons of sugar everyday. This can result in a lot of problems in the long run. Have a goal in mind and reduce the amount of sugar you consume based on this amount. If you aim to take only 15 teaspoons of sugar then do not have any sugary substances after that quota is done. This does not just include desserts, but fruit spreads, jams, soda, breakfast cereals and so on. Keep reducing the quota as you progress from say 15 teaspoons to 10 teaspoons.

7. Remove sugar from regular recipes. If your cooking requires you to add sugar simply don't put any into the pan. Most recipes like soups, casseroles, sauces and so on call for some amount of sugar. Also cuisines like Thai

cuisine, Chinese cuisine and some forms of Indian cuisine, have higher amounts of sweet content added to balance the dish. Either avoid adding sugars or sweeteners into these dishes or simply stop taking these cuisines all together. Avoid using tomato sauce or any other sauce that contains sugars added in them.

8. While buying any substances or consuming any type of food remember to check for any forms of hidden sugars and avoid these products accordingly. Read food labels and only go for substances that have little to no sugars. Usually substances like cough syrups and other types of medications also have copious amounts of sugar in them. Ketchup also contains huge amounts of sugars. Though these may seem like very less sugars, they can contribute to your sugar addiction. Hence it is best to avoid such products.

9. When looking for breakfast cereals, choose the cereals with the lowest amount of sugars in them. The healthy cornflakes that you see on shelves are usually packed with high amounts of sugars that can make you fat and cause disorders. A good way to check for the right type of cereals for you to eradicate your sugar addiction is to opt for those with less than 8 grams of sugar per serving. Alternately it is ideal to consume substances like oatmeal, which do not contain sugars. If the taste is not palpable and you do require more sugar opt to add cut fruits or dried fruits into your breakfast cereal.

10. Do not substitute artificial sweeteners in place of sugars. Artificial sweeteners do little to eradicate your sugar craving. Sugar craving is mostly sweet craving and artificial sweeteners do just this. They feed into your sweet craving. Artificial sweeteners and sugar substitutes often

lead to obesity. Reduce the amount of sugar in your diet. Instead of using artificial sweeteners and sugary substitutes opt for healthier options like honey and coconut syrups. You can also opt for fruit syrups but ensure they are organic and do not contain added sugar. If they do happen to, buy the one with the least amount of added sugars.

Chapter 6

Medications & Supplements

The antibiotic approach is one of the most used techniques for the treatment of SIBO. The approach targets the bacterial overgrowth in a head-on manner with the use of antibiotic drugs, with findings achieving 91% success in eradicating SIBO. The primary drugs used for this purpose are Xifaxan & Neomycin. These are non-absorbable drugs, meaning they stay in the intestines and don't risk the body with side effects like urinary tract infections. They are chosen especially for this task due to their property of specificity, which allows them to be triggered whenever they are needed.

There are 3 outstanding dosage options for Xifaxan, which may be used for all types of SIBO. Neomycin can help compliment the drug in cases where SIBO is accompanied by constipation but in case of diarrhea, Xifaxan alone is enough. The dosage options for Xifaxan & Neomycin are as follows:

➢ Xifaxan:

    i.   1600mg/day for 10 days,

ii.   1200 mg/day for 14 days,

iii.   1200 mg/day for 19 days with 5g/day Partially Hydrolyzed Guar gum

➤ Xifaxan plus Neomycin:

i.   1600mg/day plus 1000mg/day, both for 10 days,

The drugs must be used in accordance with the advice given by your doctor. During the first few days of this treatment, you might suffer from more gas discomfort and diarrhea therefore, it is important to reduce the amount of carbohydrates in your daily diet. Patients of irritable bowel syndrome or those on anti-depressants must continue with the treatment for a long-time until symptoms ease up.

After this antibiotic treatment is completed, the subsequent muscular disturbances are treated using low doses of erythromycin or naltrexone every night before sleeping. Erythromycin is a commonly used antibiotic with properties similar to a hormone responsible for stimulating muscle activity in the small intestine. As medication is needed for a long period of time to prevent recurrence of the SIBO, those allergic to erythromycin must take Align Probiotic on a nightly basis. If both the drugs are ineffective then doses of Xifaxan need to be prescribed by your doctor.

Stomach Acid:

Another way in which SIBO can be treated is by normalizing the amount of stomach acid & enzymes. For this, you will need to take the hydrochloric acid test first which will determine the amount of Bentaine HCL you need BUT first you must be absolutely sure that you don't have a history of stomach ulcers; if this is the case then skip this treatment.

To perform, take a 450 mg dosage of the drug along with pepsin before a meal. If you notice no scorching at all, then increase the intake to 2 capsules. Keep increasing the capsules until a mild scorching sensation is felt, upon which reduce the dose by 1 capsule. For many people, a dose between lower than 3 capsules does the trick quite easily. If burning sensation is caused due to just a single capsule then you either have too little acid or the reflux you suffer is too severe for any medication; you'll have to hold off until it's under control. Moreover, the more proteins you consume, the more HCL you'll need, so keep varying your doses in accordance with the size of your meals. If extreme gastrointestinal problems are what you're suffering from then taking a food enzyme that has both pancreatic enzymes plus HCL will be your best bet.

In less than 6 months you might start feeling some warmth in your stomach at the same dosage levels; when this starts to happen then decrease your Betaine intake.

Next, digestive bitters which are essential for aiding in secretions & stimulations in the small intestine. Bitters are not only good at stimulating HCL, but they also cause the release of bile from the gallbladder and enzymes from the pancreas. Bitter are most effective when taken 20 minutes before a meal along with one large glass of water. A taste of salt along with the water is also helpful as it provides the necessary chloride for the drug. You must consider the following digestive bitters:

Angostura bitters

   i.   Swedish Bitters

   ii.   Organic Bitters

iii.   Digestive Bitters

iv.   Grape Bitters

Bitters must be laid off if you suffer from digestive atrophy meaning dry mucus membranes, which can be diagnosed through dry & shriveled tongue.

SIBO can also become a cause to leaky gut, which means damage to the linings of the small intestine. To cure this, take zinc supplements for a month, 200 mg daily plus a probiotic capsule like the previously mentioned Align or Flora-Q under your doctor's guidance. You may also need to take vitamin & mineral supplements due to bacterial presence that may have resulted in early absorption of vital nutrients by the bacteria. Taking vitamin B12, A, D, E & K, magnesium, calcium, copper & iron, can rectify common deficiencies.

Lastly, restrictions on artificial sugars can also help the patient in the long-term as it would reduce recurrence of SIBO. Try to avoid all products, natural or synthetic that are high on sugar to beat this disease once and for all.

Chapter 7
Herbal Treatment

There is no denying the fact that antibiotics have been one of the most useful advancement in modern medicine; they have saved God-knows how many lives and made life for the common man quite easy. But just like every other synthetic medical innovation, antibiotics aren't perfect, they have brought along several risks as well. Sometimes antibiotics can't be the right technique for treatment and therefore an alternative must be used instead. Very effective as well as purely natural alternatives are herbal anti-microbes for the treatment of Small Intestinal Bacterial Overgrowth.

I've prepared a list of common side effects associated with drugs used to treat SIBU. These are:

Drug	Side-effect
Rifaximin	Bloating, stomach pain, gas, headache, dizziness, mild insomnia
Neomycin	Irritation, nausea, vomiting
Metronidazole	Back pain, confusion, agitation, weakness

Therefore, if you wish to avoid these side effects, it's better to choose herbal anti-microbes over them.

Grapefruit Seed Extract:

Grapefruit Seed Extract or GSE is a natural remedy for several health problems and is a common ingredient in self-help products; it is widely available in supplement form as well. GSE possess several properties one of which is being an antioxidant, due to a substance known as naringenin. It acts as an antimicrobial agent and destroys several harmful microorganisms in the body. Here are the properties of the extract that prove its worth in many ways:

i. Antibacterial agent – GSE is very effective against bacteria that dwell in the body including the gut, which means extra bacteria in the small intestine would get diminished.

ii. Pancreatitis – A study published in the Journal of Physiology Pharmacy showed that GSE was protective against inflammation in the pancreas.

The research on the extract is still ongoing but some evidence does indicate that intake of naringenin found in GSE can reduce inflammation, bacteria and boost overall health of a person. Having said that, I must say that many supplements available in the market are mixed with synthetic materials so when buying a supplement make sure it's of a trusted brand or one that your doctor recommends you.

Oregano Oil Capsules:

Oregano oil is an extremely popular natural remedy, available in supplement form, known for its antioxidant, antifungal, antibacterial and antiviral properties. So far it has been found that oregano oil capsules can help against:

i. Colitis – a type of inflammatory bowel disease (remember?), which can come as a consequence of Small Intestinal Bowel Syndrome.

ii. Candida – a type of yeast that dwells in the digestive tract causing infections if it goes unchecked. Oregano oils can help against these infections.

iii. Bacteria – Oregano capsules have the ability to kill bacteria that cause dysentery.

It is advised that you use this remedy with the advice of your health care provider.

Goldenseal:

Goldenseal is a historic herb now used commonly in the market for treating a variety of health problems. Originally Native Americans used it for the treatment of digestive problems, skin disorders, liver condition and diarrhea. Goldenseal attained worldwide success in the 1800s and since then has become the subject much research. It is available in supplement form and is also available as an ointment for wounds.

Goldenseal is a bitter that stimulates the flow of bile that results in benefits for the gut, namely healthy intestines and stomach.

Olive leaf extract:

A natural substance as the name indicates the extract is obtained from leaves of the olive plant and possesses several compounds that have a positive effect on health. One of these compounds known as oleuropein possesses antibacterial, antioxidant and immunity boosting properties. Not only this but olive leaf extracts can allow beneficial bacteria to grow which means it acts as a probiotic as well. This was found when olive leaf extract was added to yogurt cultures; there was no effect on the yogurt meaning that the bacteria were unharmed. Olive leaf extract is beneficial for the gut due to its antibiotic plus probiotic property that kills harmful bacteria but retains the essential ones, a property vital for the cure of Small Intestinal Bacterial Overgrowth.

Furthermore, it has been found that bacteria can get resilient to artificial antibiotics, meaning you can continue dozing off antibiotics but there will be no effect on them. But it has been found that even though bacteria can form resistance to traditional drugs, they are helpless against natural antimicrobials like the Olive Leaf Extract, resulting in a sure shot against harmful microorganisms.

Just 5 drops of the miracle extract would do wonders for your intestinal health.

Dill:

Dill is a popular flavoring agent that has been used throughout 2000 years of history. It has a calming effect on both the nervous and the digestive system. It is a natural diuretic, antibacterial and a pancreatic stimulant; the last 2 properties of Dill make it ideal for the cure of SIBO.

Other natural products that may prove useful in the quest against SIBO include:

- Wormwood,
- Brucea javanica,
- Rhizome,
- The leaf Yarrow,
- French Tarragon,
- Thyme,
- Pau d'arco

You must also know that I am not making a hollow claim on the effectiveness of natural antimicrobials. A study published in the Global Advances in Health & Medicine in 2014 proved that antimicrobials were as much effective as antibiotics for the treatment of SIBO. In the study 104 patients of SIBO were treated with either 1200mg of Rifaximin or with a mixture of herbs for a period of 4 weeks. After the specified period of time it was found that 46% of the patients who were treated naturally had successfully beaten off SIBO whereas only 34% of the Rifaximin group was cured. Just so you want to know the herbal combinations were one of the following, twice a day.

1. Dysbiocide & FC Cidal,

2. Candibactin AR & Candibactin BR

Don't give up, utilize every resource you have and you are bound to beat the condition.

Chapter 8

Specific Carbohydrate Diet

All dietary treatments that you go through to cure Small Intestinal Bacterial Growth will be based, more or less on the same concept: to reduce the sources of food on which bacteria thrive. The diets usually seek to keep the person healthy but starve the bacteria, which is a clever trick. It has been found through various studies that bacteria thrive on carbohydrates so every diet that claims to cure SIBO must meet this requirement before any other; the only type of carbohydrate that bacteria don't like is insoluble fiber so no need to lower its intake. There are a number of diets that can help in the treatment of SIBO, including:

- ✓ The Gut & Psychology Syndrome Diet,
- ✓ The Low FODMAPs Diet,
- ✓ The Specific Carbohydrate Diet,
- ✓ The Paleo Diet,
- ✓ A combination of Diets,

After reading the requirement for bacteria to live, it must've been instantly clear why I named the chapter after the Specific Carbohydrate Diet. The reason is simple; the Specific Carbohydrate Diet is basically build around the concept of different types of Carbohydrates and how they affect our body, therefore due to the specificity of the diet, it has been chosen as the best treatment for SIBO.

The Specific Carbohydrate Diet was created by the famous pediatrician Sidney Haas and has proven great relief for people suffering from many diseases, mostly of the gut including Crohn's disease, Cystic Fibrosis, IBS, Diarrhea, etc. The diet is based on the fact that dented intestinal walls along with overgrowth of bacteria cause a vicious cycle that takes a toll on the body's overall health. The diet aims to restrict free-hand carbohydrates access, which as mentioned earlier are the diet of these bacteria! By doing this, the body's inner ecology is restored and it gets on the path to rehabilitation.

The strict yet very useful grain-free, sucrose-free & lactose-free regimen combats yeasts as well as bacterial infections in the body, in this case the small intestine by cutting off the microorganism food supply. This can be done only when the foods eaten are low in carbohydrates; or they should contain monosaccharides that are absorbed quickly by the body reducing the chances of bacteria consuming it. A list of allowed food products is given later but first you should understand the concept of how it all works.

First of all, you should know that there are 3 basic types of sugars:

i.   Simple sugars or monosaccharides,

ii.   Disaccharides, e.g. sucrose, lactose,

iii.   Polysaccharides, e.g. starches

Now, when you consume any food, the body must break it down to monosaccharides if it is to be absorbed into the bloodstream. If the body fails to do so, the real trouble begins then.

Of all the components there are of food, carbohydrates are the most vital ones for bacteria involved in intestinal disorders. The Specific Carbohydrate Diet works by limiting the availability of these carbs to the microorganisms; if carbs aren't digested, they do not get absorbed and you know what that means. They stay in the intestinal tract multiplying colonies of various bacteria. This multiplication is often followed by intestinal disorders like formation of acids or toxins harmful for the small intestine. So you see that bacteria themselves aren't harmful, but the effect & influence they have on the body is. Now, once these bacteria start to multiply they destroy the enzymes that are present on the intestinal surface causing a carbohydrate absorption blockade. At this particular point, the body senses danger and starts to produce abnormal amounts of mucus to lubricate the walls of the intestine in an effort to reduce irritation caused by the acids, toxins and semi-digested food bits along with carbohydrates.

I'm guessing that at this point you might be getting the concept behind lactose intolerance as well. Lactose intolerance is a condition that is branded by the lack of enzymes that are responsible for breaking down lactose into monosaccharides. Lactose itself is a disaccharide meaning that it can't be absorbed by the digestive system; this means that gut bacteria feed off it that causes overgrowth. The same scenario can be extended to all disaccharides as well as polysaccharides, therefore, all types of

complex carbohydrates are restricted by the diet in order to bring down the symptoms of SIBO.

The Specific Carbohydrate Diet states that not all types of carbohydrates fall prey to traps set by bacteria; simple carbohydrates can still be absorbed in the body while keeping bacteria cut off from any food source. With the passage of time the number of bacteria starve off & die and with them their toxins diminish as well. Finally, the cycle stops and the mucus-producing cells stop the excessive flow of mucus, improving the digestion & absorption of carbohydrates. Moreover, the diet also promotes the use of probiotic or fermented products like yogurt, as the gut still needs healthy bacteria to function properly.

The Specific Carbohydrate Diet therefore corrects the process of absorption that allows the nutrients including carbohydrates to enter into the bloodstream through a proper & healthy channel. This leads to a re-strengthened immune system that is better prepared for a bacterial overgrowth attack this time.

Safety of the Specific Carbohydrate Diet:

You might have some doubts about the diet, which I'm pretty sure would be answered in this section. SCD has been in existence for more than sixty years and has brought relief to thousands of sufferers of SIBO. The diet is way more nutritious compared to common diets like the Standard American Diet. Moreover, in no manner is SCD a drug! It has an efficient cost/benefit ratio with the greatest one being a life free of diseases; if anything, it decreases the cost of food by reducing manufactured and processed items from your meal. Many people who have followed the Specific Carbohydrate Diet have developed an opinion that money is not better than health and therefore, extra effort to fulfill your snack-cravings in a healthy manner shouldn't be avoided. Give the following a little thought: by spending a little more on the preparations of foods, you will be saving so many costly medical bills, especially if you don't have insurance. Therefore, SCD is your best option to treat Small Intestinal Bacterial Overgrowth and uplift the gut's health in general.

SCD is not a low-carb diet; instead it is a specific diet that allows certain foods while prohibiting others. If the diet is to be low at something, it is processed food products, as it requires a lot of food items to be prepared in the conventional way. I've prepared a list of foods that are allowed & disallowed when on the diet:

Disallowed:

1. Sugars – foods that contain sucrose, fructose or any other type of processed sugar.

2. Veggies – All canned vegetables, all grains like wheat, corn, oats, barley, rice, etc. and some legumes i.e. bean sprouts, chick peas, soybeans, mung beans, garbanzo beans and fava beans are not allowed.

3. Starchy foods – like yams, parsnips and potatoes are not permitted.

4. Meats – All canned meats are prohibited,

5. Dairy – Each and every type of milk variations are forbidden, whether its skim, whole, 1%, chocolate, etc. Cheeses that contain high percentage of lactose are also to be laid off; these include, Mozzarella, cream cheese, cottage cheese, feta, cheese spreads, etc. Along with these commercially available yogurts are also not allowed as they contain high amounts of lactose.

6. Misc. – other foods include bread, canola oil, mayonnaise, cocoa, candy, ice cream, margarine, whey powder, baking powder and mixed nuts.

Allowed:

The diet does not restrict the quantity of any food.

1.   Sugars – the only allowed sugar products are honey, brown rice syrup and molasses. It is vital that you use these products with caution as some people can develop a reaction to them.

2.   Veggies – almost all vegetables in fresh, frozen or cooked form are allowed, e.g. broccoli, artichokes, beets, cauliflower, cabbage, sprouts, spinach, etc. In case of diarrhea, raw vegetables must be avoided.

3.   Meats – unprocessed meats like chicken, turkey, beef, fish, lamb, eggs, etc. are allowed.

4.   Dairy – natural cheeses with exception to those mentioned in the previous section are allowed. Homemade yogurt is also encouraged due to its probiotic content.

5.   Fruits – most of the fruits are allowed including apples, olives, avocadoes, bananas, dates, berries, etc. except for seedless grapes & tomatoes because they play a part in disrupting in the regular process of digestion.

6.   Nuts – edible seeds & nuts like almonds; walnuts, filberts & pecans are allowed with the exception of cashews, macadamia nuts and pistachios as they contain harmful chemicals in their raw forms.

7.   Misc. – other foods allowed under the diet include coconut, olive, soybean and corn oil; weak tea & coffee; mustard, vinegar and juices that pack no additives.

That's it for the Specific Carbohydrate Diet; it you follow the diet in a strict manner there is a 75% chance of success after which you may switch back to a free-hand diet. The way in which the diet works has been explained and should be enough to convince you that this is the best diet for treating SIBO. But if you have other things in mind then you may use any of the other diets listed at the start of the chapter.

The next few chapters' deals with food replacements in detail so if you plan on following strict dietary guidelines then I highly recommend reading the next few chapters.

Maria Lexington

Chapter 9
Paleo Diet

Paleo diet is commonly also known as Paleolithic diet and this diet is one, which is based on the foods that were consumed by early men. The diet includes substances like meats, nuts and berries and avoids substances like milk, which had not been found out. It is based on the nutritional requirement of early cavemen and takes a spin off on their food. In this kind of diet, it is believed that the nutritional requirement of the beings of those era were based on the food that was available and hence the nutritional needs of the modern man does not change and would still comply with his Paleolithic ancestors. Advocates of the Paleo diet believe that the human metabolism has not been able to adapt to substances like dairy and therefore could only eat substances since the discovery of agriculture. In it there is more meat and protein based items that are consumed. These include seafood and animal products. There is also a higher fat intake. Lesser carbohydrates in consumed and lots of fibrous vegetables and fruits are consumed. Substances like dairy products, processed oils, salt, sugar, legumes and grains are not consumed.

It is widely prescribed today for those who have troubles pertaining to the gut including the leaky gut syndrome, IBS and SIBO. Leaky gut syndrome and other gut related problems can cause further complications like inflammatory bowel disease, chronic fatigue, diabetes, rashes, and mental disorders and so on. It is important to note that every food that you do consume has some reaction in your gut. Some substances can cause problems in the gut and cause reactions such as gut permeability. This can make the food enter the bloodstream and this in turn will create antibodies. On a long-term basis it can even cause autoimmune diseases.

In a Paleo diet it is ideal to consume substances that are rich in probiotics like fermented vegetables, sauerkraut, yogurt and so on. The gut contains several microorganisms and these microorganisms can cause trouble when they aren't balanced by healthy bacteria. These healthy bacteria are found in fermented probiotic substances. It is also important to consume substances like bone broth and fermented substances. These are rich in components like gelatin, glutamine and other substances that help in repairing the lining of the gut.

There are several benefits of following a Paleo diet. It results in healthy cell formation. This is because it contains high amounts of saturated fats and these fats are important components of cells. Thus, the saturated fat content in the Paleo diet can account for high amounts of cell generation. This is especially important for those with the leaky gut syndrome. The lining of the gut can get severely damaged and by having a Paleo diet you encourage the cells to regenerate and this will help in healing the lining of the gut. Alternately it can also help in soothing the inflammation. Another major advantage of the Paleo diet is that it accounts for the growth of muscles instead of fat. This is because of the high protein content in the food. The high protein content found in it can account for the basic building blocks of our body. These protein help in repairing the gut and repairing any damaged tissues. They also help in purifying the blood and bones. With Paleo diet, you increase the metabolism of your gut. This is because, sugars, processed foods and other refined substances can account to having a bad gut. These cause inflammation of the gut and create problems in your digestive tracts. This is further aggravated by lots of stress.

The Paleo diet also contains all the necessary nutrients and vitamins that you require. Though it seems like you are eliminating a lot of substances, you gain adequate amounts of nutrients and enzymes that are required for your general immunity. It also contains huge amounts of vegetables and these are often very good for health as they are loaded with natural sugars that are easy to breakdown. They also help in repairing your body and rejuvenating it. Thus it also accounts for better digestion and absorption. This is because the diet is something that is a constituent of your genes. Our ancestors have been taking this type of diet for centuries and hence you are naturally able to process these types of foods a lot better. They also reduce inflammation. Inflammation can often lead to cardiovascular problems. When inflammation is reduced, there are fewer chances of complications occurring. The other advantage of Paleo diet is that it recognizes your body's needs and does not pay attention to your addictions. The body gets desensitized when fed copious amounts of sugars and refined substances and hence starts to malfunction. Thus the Paleo diet increases the insulin sensitivity of your body.

Tips to follow a Paleo diet

Paleo diet is often considered hard to follow and there are several rules and regulations including restrictions in this type of diet. In this section we explore the various ways through which you can follow a Paleo diet.

1. Paleo diet is a diet, which is high in fat. It is ideal to opt for fats that are good for health. Use fruits and vegetables and organic oils to achieve this as opposed to sugary substances, which are the wrong type of fats. This diet is also moderate on proteins so it is a good idea to consume animal proteins. You can also take fruits and vegetables that are high in proteins. Try not to load up on carbohydrate rich foods like grains.

2. Take substances that are rich in saturated fats. Saturated fats are beneficial for health. Saturated fats are found in substances like clarified butter, butter and coconut oil. You can also take lard, goose fat, duck fat, beef tallow and so on. You can also use nut oils like macadamia oils and drizzle them in soups and salads as dressing. You can also use olive oil and avocado oil for cooking instead. These fats help in increased liver health and increases metabolism and immunity. They also help in proper brain signaling and increase the efficiency of the body.

3. Eat bigger amounts of animal protein and remember to eat good sources of them as well. Animal proteins include substances like red meat, pork, eggs, poultry, organs like kidney, heart, liver, seafood and so on. It is also ideal to consume the fatty parts of these animals. The animal protein should also contain animal fat, which is an important component of Paleo diet. You can use the bones and the parts you don't generally consume in making stocks. You can also consume the meat that is located or stuck on the bones. These are usually very rich in nutrients and help in digestion.

4. Have copious amounts of fresh vegetables. You can also have them frozen as well. Pick vegetables and have them raw or cooked and drizzled with some fat. You can look for substances that are not starchy like sweet potatoes and yams and these do not contain poisonous or high levels of carbohydrates. These carbohydrates are easy t breakdown by your digestive system. Top these with some olive oil or any nut oil. You can also top with some saturated fats like duck fat, lard and so on.

5. Also make it a point to consume moderate amounts of fruits and nuts. Ensure that the fruits that you are going to consume are low in sugar like berries. These are usually high in substances like antioxidants, which are extremely important at neutralizing the toxic substances in your body. Nuts are also really good for you ensure that you take nuts that are rich in substances like omega fatty acids like omega 3. Do not take substances like macadamia nuts as they have polysaturated fats, which can harm you. Also avoid nuts that are high in omega 6 like peanuts. Do not load up on these if you do have autoimmune diseases.

6. Choose organic meat over anything else. Opt for meats that are pasture raised and grass fed. Also choose meat from environmentally friendly farms. This will reduce impurities in the system. You can also choose the lean cuts that don't have much fat in it. These cuts can be drizzled with fatty substances like coconut oil, ghee or butter to ensure that they give the adequate nutrients. Also when using vegetables choose those vegetables that are locally produced. You can go in for seasonal varieties also but ensure that they are organically grown.

7. Reduce the consumption of having grains, legumes and cereals from your diet. Wheat, oats, barley, soy, pinto

beans and so on are not advisable. Therefore do not take them. This is because these foods can cause inflammation and can cause further complications in the gut. Another important thing to remember is to avoid taking substances like gluten substances. They can also weaken your immune system and give you irregular bowel movements.

8. Get rid of all vegetable oils. It is best to avoid these in both varieties including hydrogenated vegetables oils as well as party hydrogenated vegetable oils. These also include corn oil, peanut oil, canola oil and margarine. Opt to cook with ghee, clarified butter, and butter and duck fats instead. You can use substances like olive oil for dressing and it goes with avocado oil too. It is better to use them as dressing instead of cooking them. This is because refined vegetable oils ruins the fatty components of your body and creates an imbalance and they also cause inflammation.

9. Do not take substances like soft drinks, aerated substances, sweet juices and packaged fruit juices. These contain huge amounts of added sugars and preservatives, which are very harmful.

10. Do not take dairy products. You can opt for butter but it is best to avoid dairy products. This is because dairy products can trigger gut reactions and can lead to complication in digestion. You can however have fermented dairy products like yogurt instead. These contain good bacteria that are good for the gut.

11. Break your meals into smaller meals and consume them. Do not skip meals and it is better if you eat when you are hungry rather than eating at set time frames.

12. Try to avoid stressful activities. Get adequate rest and sleep for a good 8 hours a day. Keep a strict sleep schedule and follow this. Wake up at a set time everyday and go to sleep at a set time everyday. Stress is a huge cause of problems in the gut. In fact people with higher amounts of stress acquire gut related problems.

13. Remember to exercise. When you exercise it is important to not over do it. Keep your exercises short and intense. Take a brisk walk and opt for quick exercises instead of those that take time.

14. Ensure you get lots of sunshine to load up on vitamin D. Vitamin D naturally reduces inflammation. It also is excellent to heal and soothe damaged parts. Vitamin D also increases your metabolism and helps in increasing your immunity. Take lots probiotics as well. Remove substances that contain huge amounts of iodine and magnesium in your diet. Opt for taking smaller amounts of these.

Maria Lexington

Chapter 10

GAPS Diet

The GAPS diet is short for Gut and Psychology Syndrome Diet and is a comprehensive diet that was formulated by Dr. Natasha Campbell-McBride. The GAPS diet begins with an introductory diet after which the whole diet is prescribed. This form of diet is used to treat those with acute digestive disorders and symptoms like bloating, constipation, diarrhea, abdominal pain and so on. The Introductory diet is used to relieve the system of these symptoms and heal the digestive tract. It is very useful in eradicating the symptoms effectively without the use of any medications. It is also recommended for those with bugs in their stomach and frequent stomach problems. The introductory diet usually gives a background and allows the body to adjust to the diet. Even the introductory diet is only initiated in stages to avoid malfunction and discomfort.

In cases of constipation, instead of using laxatives, this diet prescribes juices and concoction, which will relieve constipation. Freshly pressed juices are introduced to relieve this and some of them are substances like carrot juice. In fact, start your day with a glass of carrot juice along with some cod liver oil. The enzymes present in carrot juice will help in the production of bile juice. The lack of production of bile juice causes constipation in many cases. The lack of bile juices causes fats to become insoluble. Therefore they react with the salts in the foods and form soaps, which can cause constipation. Avoid dairy products as they too cause constipation.

Food allergies and certain foods can be rendered intolerable by people. In these cases the GAPS introductory diet helps in reducing inflammation and can heal their gut. These foods can cause a syndrome called the leaky gut where the lining of the gut is damaged by the abnormal presence of bacterial flora in the gut. Therefore the nutrients present in the foods do not get absorbed properly due to the perforations in the lining of the gut and this can cause the onset of antibodies. This can damage the immune system. The damaged lining of the gut only partially absorbs the food and this can cause abnormal reactions both slow and fast. Abnormal digestion can also cause more complications and can lead to further food allergies. Food tests for allergies have also been quite ineffective and they usually come positive for every food tested. Therefore until the lining of the gut wall is fixed and there are no faulty food passages in the system, there will not be an effective relief for food digestion. Therefore the introductory diet does just this. Once the gut wall is properly healed, the foods tend to get properly digested and absorbed.

Those who do not have adverse symptoms of IBS and have very mild food intolerances and mild digestive problems can go through the introductory diet and can get instant relief. It is very important to follow the introductory diet and then the whole diet because the body needs to adjust and comply with the sudden restriction and introduction of certain foods. Thus the gut will get optimized in this process. Not following the introductory diet can lead to long-term problems and lead to further digestive complications.

There are instances where you can directly go to the complete GAPS diet, in these cases it is important to note that about 80 to 85 per cent of the items that you do consume should be made out of meats like eggs, fish and also fermented dairy, and vegetables. Fruits and baked items must not be consumed for a while and it can then be introduced in small amounts. For instance, you can snack on some baked goods or fruits in between meals. However they should not be consumed as a part of main meals and they can get incorporated only after a few weeks. Stews, homemade meat stock, and foods that have natural fats can be consumed and should be staple foods you eat.

Now when coming to the introductory food, it is important to check for any insensitivity towards foods. The introductory GAPS diet introduces dairy earlier than the complete GAPS diet and it is for this purpose to check if you are tolerable towards dairy. In the section below we look at the introductory GAPS diet and how to implement it.

For the introduction diet, start your day with some water. You can opt for either filtered water or even mineral water. The water should be lukewarm or slightly warm. Cold water can aggravate the gut and cause it to malfunction. Alternately you can take some probiotic drinks. Now the introductory diet is introduced in stages. In the first stage, the main symptoms of diarrhea, constipation, and abdominal pain will subside and you can check this by introducing new foods that were restricted. If the symptoms start to rise again then the gut has not been healed completely and it is best to avoid the food. Continue with the old regiment and try again in a few days. There are several foods that can cause allergies and food intolerances. In these cases it is ideal to do a sensitivity test for the food.

Sensitivity test can be done by taking a little bit of the food that you think you are sensitive towards and place it on the inside of your wrist. If the food happens to be in a solid form then it is best to mash it a little bit and mix it with some water. The food sensitivity test should be done before you go to bed. Place the tiny particle of food on the inside of your wrist and let it dry. Go to sleep and check if there are any spots or any red blisters on that spot. If there are then avoid the food and continue with the diet. Try this a few days later to check your progress and then when there are no spots of blisters you can start introducing these foods onto your diet in small quantities.

So the first stage is comprised of homemade meat or fish stock. Meat and fish are rich in proteins and these proteins are the building blocks of the body. They help to repair damaged tissues and even help in cell regeneration. These will in turn heal and repair the leaky gut syndrome and reduce the perforations in the gut. They are also soothing and help in eradicating the inflammation of the gut. In fact, fish stock has been used for over several centuries as a relief for digestive disorders. While using fish stock it is important not to use the fish stocks you get in markets. These include the stock granules and cubes that contain high amounts of preservatives. They are also processed foods and the acidity regulators and other substances can do more harm than good. Other stocks like chicken stock can also be used. Chicken stock is considered to be a remedy for upset stomach and therefore can be a good starting point. It is a good idea to make your own stock at home. To do this you will require the bones, joints and the meat that is situated on the bones of the animal. You can choose chicken, parts of the chicken, goose or duck and other inexpensive meats to make the stock. However ensure you incorporate the bones and the joints when making any stock as these are highly healing in nature and the substances in them are the ones that can give you immediate relief.

You can get the bones of the meat from the butcher. Simply ask him to cut the bones in half and this will enable you to get maximum benefits due to the bone marrow. Take a large pan with water in it and add the bones, meats and the joints. You can add salt if you want and some black peppercorns according to your taste. Let it boil and cover and let it simmer for a few hours. This will extract the flavors and the natural healing ingredients found in the meat. You can make fish stock the same way. Simply toss the bones, tails, and heads of the fish and repeat the same process. After 2 to 3 hours is complete, drain by removing the bones. If the bones have some meat sticking to them then you can use this meat, as they are rich in regenerative tissues. You can even add them in soups, dishes and even salads.

Bang the bones of the meat while they are still warm on a thick surface and you will be able to extract the bone marrow out of the bones. The tissues that surround the bones and bone marrow are rich in enzymes that are soothing for the stomach and the gut. Consume them as they help in increasing the efficiency of the immune system. These tissues can be frozen and preserved up to a week to consume. A person with IBS can consume this meat stock along with his or her meals. You can also give him or her to consume after or before the meals. When serving these stocks remember not to microwave these as the radiation caused by microwave strips the stocks from the essential ingredients. It is best to use a stove for heating the stock. The fat in the stock is the key at healing the gut and helps in tissue formation. You can also add some probiotic food or substances into these stocks to help accelerate the healing process and allow good bacteria to be formed.

In the first stage you can also make the person who is suffering from IBS to consume homemade soups that contain homemade fish or meat stocks. You can look up some recipes online or stick to making basic soups using the ingredients around your house. Add some meat stock into a pan and add chopped vegetables like onions, leeks, broccoli, carrots and so on. Do not use very fibrous vegetables and stick to combinations of vegetables that you are not sensitive towards. Cabbage and celery are very fibrous and should be avoided at this stage. Let the vegetables simmer for about half an hour and any vegetables that have fibrous parts like stems and so on should be removed. Skin of the pumpkins and seeds of squashes, stalks of cauliflowers and so on must be removed because of their fibrous content. Let the vegetables cook well and you can add garlic at this stage, let it boil for a minute or so and then turn the gas off. You can also blend the components of the soup or leave it as it is. Add some probiotic substances into the soup to accelerate the process of cell growth. Drink this soup along with the tissues that were stuck to the bones of the meat.

Probiotics are very important and they should be introduced to the person suffering from gut related problems from the initial stages. Probiotic foods can be both vegetable based as well as dairy based. It is best to test for food sensitivity before using these probiotic substances in your meals. You can even introduce them in small quantities and then incorporate large amounts. For instance it is a good idea to start with a few teaspoons of the probiotic substance for about a week and then increase it to a few more and so on. You can do this until you are able to add a few teaspoons of probiotic substances into your meals. You can also use yogurt or kefir if you are responding positively to the probiotic substances.

If you are sensitive to dairy then you can use alternative probiotic foods like juice of fermented vegetables, sauerkraut and so on. When adding probiotic substances to your meals it is important to not add them when the meal is too hot. This is because the heat in the food can kill the good bacteria in probiotic foods rendering them inefficient. Ensure you take some ginger tea between your meals. You can make ginger tea by grating some ginger and adding it to some boiling water. Cover the pan with a lid and let it boil for about 4 minutes so that all the enzymes and remedying properties of the ginger root are extracted onto the water. You can add honey to this mixture and drink this tea.

When it comes to the next stage, it is important to continue with the items that you were having in stage 1. It is important to continue taking foods like soups that contain bone marrows and tissues of the bones. Meat stock and ginger tea are also to be incorporated along with some probiotic substances. Keep adding substances like fermented vegetables, yogurt, kefir, sauerkraut and so on. To these foods you can add raw egg yolk. You can take some organic raw egg yolks along with your meat stock or soups. Start with an egg yolk a day and you can increase this amount by adding more egg yolks. You can do this by adding an egg yolk to every meal. When you have gained tolerance for the egg yolks, you can add soft-boiled eggs. Ensure that the egg whites are cooked and the yolk is still runny. Add them into soups and increase this quantity. Try doing a sensitivity test if you are concerned about problems. They require little digestion so they usually aren't problematic. They also give abundant nutrition and increase metabolism. Ensure that the eggs you take are organic and are fresh.

Also at this stage you can start adding substances like stews and casseroles into your meals. These should be made of vegetables or meats and it is best to avoid using spices in their preparation. Instead opt for fresh herbs like coriander and parsley. Ensure the fat content that is present in these meals are high, this is because the fats present in animals have remedying properties that can help you recover faster. Add probiotic substances to all your servings. With every stage and with every food tolerance it is a good idea to increase the amount of yogurt and kefir you consume. You can also increase the amount of fermented vegetables and sauerkraut. At this point, once tolerance is established you start with fermented meats like fermented fish. Have a little bit a day and start to increase once you are more tolerable towards these. You should also add a teaspoon of ghee to your meals by starting slow and then increasing. Ensure the ghee is homemade, as this will not have any preservatives.

When total tolerance has been established and you have no problems with regards to food sensitivities you can move onto the third stage. In this stage it is imperative to carry on consuming all the foods that you were consuming in the previous two stages. Now you start consuming ripe avocados. Simply mash ripe avocados and add them to the soups and dishes. Start with a few teaspoons and then gradually increase the number of teaspoons of avocado. You can also start consuming pancakes. Ensure that you consume one and once you are confident enough start increasing the amount of pancakes consumed. It is best to make your pancakes using pure ingredients like any nut butter like almond, peanut or walnut, organic eggs and some vegetable like squash or marrow. Ensure the vegetable is mashed and blended using a food processor. Make your batter using these ingredients and fry your pancake using some ghee. You can also use some duck or goose fat.

Instead of using just soft-boiled eggs and egg yolks you can now take your eggs scrambled. Accompany scrambled eggs with some ghee, avocado and vegetables. When looking at vegetables opt for vegetables like onions for they are extremely good for the digestive tract. Use substances like duck fat or goose fat to cook the slices of the onions for a few minutes on a low heat. You can also use ghee at this point. Now you can start having pure sauerkraut and fermented vegetables. Initially you were drinking the juice of these vegetables; now start incorporating these into your diet. Start with small tiny servings like a few tablespoons after every meal. You can then start increasing once you know you can tolerate these.

When you can digest all these and you feel no discomfort you can begin with stage 4. In this stage ensure you incorporate all the previous foods in the previous stages into your diet. Do not consume fried vegetables or meat at this stage. However you can add meats that are cooked by grilling or roasting at this stage. Do not burn or char the vegetables or the meat. You can take your vegetables with sauerkraut and other fermented vegetables. Do not barbecue the vegetables or meats yet. At this stage start to incorporate cold pressed olive oil into your meals. You can take a few drops at a time and then increase it to a few tablespoons per meal. You can also start taking fresh juices. Start with a few tablespoons of carrot juice. At this stage, ensure that your juice is clear and that it is drained and filtered well. You can dilute this by adding some water or mix it in some yogurt. You can increase the quantity to a cup a day if you tolerate it. Add mint, lettuce and celery juice also but ensure that you start small. It is ideal to drink these as soon as you wake up. You can drink them in the afternoon. At this stage you can also start incorporating baked items like some bread and so on. It is a good idea to take baked items that have seeds and nuts in them like almonds or pecans and so on. Simply use nut flour, some eggs and incorporate with them some mashed squash. You can also use ghee and butter along with some salt. Take a little bit and increase the quantities, as you feel more comfortable with it.

When you are thorough and comfortable with the foods you are taking and you manage to be able to digest all these foods easily you can proceed to the next stage that is stage 5. In this stage you can take all the previous foods that you were taking. In this stage, you can start to incorporate apples in your diet. You can start slow by incorporating cooked apple or an apple puree. Simply apples and ensure they are ripe. Steam or strew the apples in boiling water until they are cooked or they become very soft. You can then mash the cooked apple and add some ghee to it. You can also add some duck fat or goose fat if you prefer. Take a few tablespoons of it and check for any reactions. If you manage to get any reactions then avoid these. If you do not experience any discomfort you can start increasing the quantities as the day's progress.

You can also add vegetables, which are raw in this stage. Take raw lettuce and some raw cucumber and incorporate these into your diet. You can also take any other soft vegetables that can be consumed raw. Watch for any reactions especially your bowel movements and passing of stools. If there are no adverse reactions you can start with more vegetables. You can gradually start incorporating other vegetables like carrots, cabbage, onions, tomatoes and so on. Previously you were taking juices of carrots, lettuce, mint and so on. Now to these juices start adding fruits but avoid taking any citrus fruits like lemons and oranges. Start with substances like apple, mango, and pineapple.

Finally you can come to the last stage, if everything you have taken so far is well tolerated and you don't face any adverse reactions to any of the substances. At this stage you can start taking substances like apple in the raw form. Start with some raw apple peels and shavings. If you are able to ingest this with no hassle then include more raw fruits. At this stage also take more honey. You can start taking cakes and other baked goods in larger quantities. You can also use more sweet products in this stage and alternately use naturally sweet substances like dried fruits. Now it is important to note that there is no particular time frame regarding the introductory diet. This is because any dietary changes or introduction of new foods can only be taken when it becomes tolerable and this can vary depending on the person. It is important to proceed to next stages only if there are no problems in the previous stage. Watch your stools and see if there is a control in diarrhea. If these start to clear up, it is a clear sign on moving to the next stage. It is also important to check for food sensitivity. If you are sensitive to certain foods avoid taking it until you become all right. After your problems disappear you should still consume soups and the meat stock. You can do this once a day. You can then proceed to the full GAPS diet once you face no problems and your basic problems are cleared.

In the full GAPS diet you should start your day with some mineral water. You can also opt for filtered water at this stage and take it with a little bit of lemon. In this stage you can have the water, hot or cold. Alternately you can also have some fresh juices either fruit or vegetable that can be diluted with water. A good tip in this point is to make a juice using apples, beetroots and carrots. Simply make the juice in a ratio of 4:1:5 and ensure that they are raw. You can also try various other combinations like cabbage, spinach, dill, basil, pineapple, grapefruit, mango and so on. Either dilute the juice using some water or simply add it to some yogurt and have it.

Ensure you get adequate sleep. With the body being constantly active it is important to ensure the body gets the right nutrients. The body goes into detoxifying mode once in a while and by drinking mineral water or drinking fresh juices you can help in this detoxifying process. During hours like 4am to 10am, the body is trying to get rid of pollutants and this is the reason one should not eat heavy meals at this time. It is best to take meals after 10am when the detoxifying process is done. It is during this time when you start to feel hungry. At this stage you can start having eggs with some sausages.

You can opt to cook these in any format and take some salads with these. Some meat and eggs can also be consumed in the morning. You can also use lots of olive oil as a dressing in all your dishes. It is best to keep the yolks uncooked while the whites of the eggs are cooked. Have a medley of vegetables and fruits like tomato, cucumber, celery and so on and sprinkles some sesame seeds. You can also use pumpkin seeds or sunflower seeds instead. When cooking sausages, use pepper and salt and avoid using herbs. Avoid buying and consuming products with MSG. It is best to ask your butcher to make pure sausages for you. You can also consume some avocados, fish or raw vegetables. It is a good idea to consume some meat stock or fish stock. Have some ginger tea also. You can also opt for pancakes that have some nuts and berries.

For lunch, opt for vegetable soup or meat soups. Have some cooked vegetables and some meat. You can use olive oil to dress them. Also have some homemade stock and for dinner you can do the same. At these points you can also use the juice of some citrus fruits like lemon or orange for dressing.

Chapter 11

FODMAP Diet

Irritable Bowel syndrome is something that affects everyone and can affect people at least once in their lives. With symptoms like acute bloating, flatulence, abdominal pain and diarrhea or constipation, it can lead to several discomfort and embarrassing situations. There are several ways through which diet can control IBS and one of the most common ways is through the low FODMAP diet. Other treatments can vary from laxatives, binding agents, medications, antibiotics and so on. Though these are also very effective, they are more short term and hence most of the people in this category have managed to get a relapse of their IBS symptoms. Australian researchers from the University of Monash came up with the low FODMAP diet, which is a dietary regiment that takes into consideration and eliminates those foods that can trigger symptoms. It has been proved to be very effective in controlling IBS. Today, the low FODMAP diet is the most widely prescribed diet in eliminating IBS across the world. This is because it encourages good bacteria growth in the gut. It must be important to note that this diet does not eliminate FODMAP completely and it is not a diet that can or should be followed throughout the life of the person. It is better to get expert advice from a dietitian or a nutritionist for those who want to take this form of diet. The time frame regarding this usually ranges from 6 weeks to 8 weeks depending upon the constitution of the person and the severity of the symptoms.

Now comes the major part as to what FODMAP is. FODMAP are a form of carbohydrates and is an acronym and it stands for Fermentable Oligo-, Di-, and Mono-saccharides And Polyols. In the diet one has to reduce the consumption of foods that contain these nutrients. Few of these carbohydrates are sugars like fructose and lactose and some are sugar alcohols like sorbitol and amnnitol. They also contain indigestible fibers like glactans and fructans. These components are naturally occurring and can be found in substances like fruits, dairy, grains, and beans and so on. Some of these components are also usually found in food preservatives and food processed products. Sugar free diabetic foods also contain huge amounts of these components in them.

The concept behind the low FODMAP diet is quite simple. Carbohydrates are present in all kinds of foods and there are several forms of carbohydrates ranging from those like starch to very simple ones like glucose. These get digested and produce energy for the body to function. Carbohydrates are also of the types where they are fibers and resistant starch and these kinds help in bowel movement and help in aiding digestion. Research has shown that there are short chains of carbohydrates, which can hinder the bowel movement and cause abnormalities leading to IBS. This is because they are not absorbed in the small intestine and they also end up getting fermented in the gut.

This fermentation process gives rise to flatulence, which can lead to other IBS related symptoms. The research regarding this has shown that out of four patients at least three patients have shown success rates with consuming the low FODMAP diet. It is not just related to treating IBS and allied symptoms; it also increases the metabolism of the gut, reduces any inflammation in the digestive tract and neutralizes any poisonous substances found in the gut. Those who have their colons removed face discomforts and problems like loose stools and infrequent bowel movements, which are taken care of by the low FODMAP diet. It is best to consult a dietitian or a nutritionist before getting into it, as this diet is usually tailor made according to a person. It must be noted that it does not completely cure IBS but it can reduce the severity of the symptoms and can reduce the medications that you take and eradicate the discomfort you feed due to IBS. In short, it lets you manage IBS.

The effect of FODMAP on the digestive tract varies depending on the type of FODMAP. Specific enzymes that are produced in the gut are required to break down the carbohydrate sugars and this can get hindered when adequate enzymes are not produces especially substances like sugar alcohols. These pull the water from the tissues around into the digestive tract and are osmotic. Fibers are foods that are fed by the bacteria in our gut and they get digested due to fermentation resulting in huge amounts of carbon dioxide produced in the gut. Therefore consuming these products in huge amounts can cause problems. It must be noted that FODMAPS are also essential as they too can foster healthy bacteria in the gut. Usually people with IBS have a lower tolerance for substances like FODMAPS. It can cause severe bloating, pain, flatulence and so on.

Foods like dairy products are most high in FODMAPS. Hence reducing the amount of dairy consumed can be a good start in getting into the low FODMAP diet. Fruits like apples, cherries, melons; mango, papaya, pears and so on contain FODMAPS in the form of fructose. Other vegetables like garlic, cabbage, asparagus, and mushrooms and so on also contain these components. Grains like wheat, barley, rye and most of the leguminous plants like soybeans are those that contain FODMAPS. Even sweeteners including natural ones like honey contain FODMAPS. They also form an important component of food coloring as well.

It might seem like a lot but there are several other substances and alternatives that can give you the same amount of nutrients without giving you the complications that come with FODMAPS. These foods can then be reintroduced in small amounts as time progresses. The advantage with the FODMAP diet is that it eliminates various components that can cause IBS and other allied digestive disorders. It is a good idea to test a few of the substances and see the reactions you get from consuming them. If you do experience symptoms then it is best to avoid these fruits and vegetables. There are times when pears and melons might work for you but beans might not. In which case getting rid or avoiding beans in your diet can lead to a healthier gut.

Chapter 12

Replacements

Sugar substitutes:

Over the last 100 years, technology and research has advanced at an unprecedented rate and almost every field of science has made equal gains. One such gain is "Sugar-substitutes"; almost everyone who suffers from sugar addiction is under a constant state of confusion as to whether he/she can use sugar substitutes and will they affect his/her health with respect to sugar addiction.

The question is a tricky one as any sugar product, whether it's natural or artificial activates the brain's reward system that makes us feel good; exactly the thing we're fighting against. However, it has been found that sugar substitutes, aspartame in particular isn't a bad idea as artificial sugars don't have as much kick when compared to natural sugars like those obtained from honey, fruits, etc. These sugar substitutes may give you part of the kick you need but don't necessarily fuel the ongoing sugar addiction.

With that being said, artificial sugars are slowly but surely taking over the commercial food industry as they can be found everywhere from soft drinks to fruit juices to sweets, etc. So are artificial sugars really that safe for human consumption that they may be included in the diet without no check & balance? It has been found that while artificial sugars do help in overcoming sugar addiction, they can give rise to a number of other problems like obesity. Other ongoing studies have also found a link between these sugars and cancer so conclusively; you should only resort to these sugars if you are suffering from too many withdrawal effects.

Vegetables:

Vegetables should top the list of foods that you consume as a measure to fill the cavity sugar deficiency leaves. Vegetables are nutritious, vitamin rich, low-calorie foods that have very little side effects, if any. The general rule that you should remember when picking up vegetables is, the greener the better. This rule applies on everyone, but has special significance for sugar addicts, as the color of the vegetable is directly proportional to its sugar content.

For the most part, vegetables are great and should be eaten to combat sugar addiction however, there are a few vegetables that are more towards the sugar spectrum and pack carbohydrates; these should be consumed in moderation or avoided as a whole. The detailed table is given below however the names of a few high carbohydrate vegetables include acorn, butternut, squash, legumes, lentils, etc. But these foods always take precedence over junk foods and other processed sugars as they have a lower tendency to trigger a sugar addiction. Nonetheless, you should be aware of the carbohydrate content of each vegetable and should make your decisions accordingly.

The table that shows the carbohydrate content of a number of vegetables is as follows. The list is arranged in ascending order and the serving size is set up at 1 cup; ideally you should consume the foods that are on the upper side of the list.

Vegetable	Carbohydrate
Endive	1.7 grams
Romanian lettuce	1.8 grams
Mushrooms	2.3 grams
Celery	3.6 grams
Pumpkin	4.2 grams
Cauliflower	5.3 grams
Spinach	7.0 grams
Tomatoes	7.0 grams
Egg plant	8.6 grams
Squash	10 grams
Broccoli	11.2 grams
Onions	16.2 grams
Artichokes	18.8 grams
Sweet potatoes	23 grams
Butternut squash	24.1 grams
Parsnips	26.5 grams
Corn	31.7 grams

Maria Lexington

Fruits:

Fruits are one of the more controversial food items that are often a point of contention for sugar addicts. Like vegetables fruits can also be high in carbohydrates and sugars especially fructose that is a natural sugar. But even with their high sugar content, there are a few reasons as to why fruits shouldn't be completely overlooked in the fight against sugar addiction.

The first and foremost reasons is that unlike drugs & alcohol that can be completely eliminated from your life, sugar cannot; it is simply impossible to never consume sugar as you live on. The only thing you can do is cut back on your sugar intake but that's it. That's where fruits come in, which provide a healthy and not-so-addicting alternative to various sugary foods. In addition, sugar packs a number of antioxidants and phytonutrients that do well for the body.

Try to consume at least 2 pieces of fruit every day and choose fruits that have lower carbohydrate content as given in the table below. Blackberries and raspberries are great for sugar-addicts but at the same time you should avoid dried fruits as they have greater sugar content to their watery counterparts.

What about fruit juices?

Try your best to avoid fruit juices especially packed ones as one big glass of sugar can contain as much sugar as 12 individual pieces. Furthermore, these juices contain added corn syrup and sucrose that makes them sweeter and even more harmful for a recovering addict. They also don't have any fiber and are thus not beneficial for gut health. All in all, avoid fruit juices and stick to raw pieces.

The table below shows the amount of carbohydrates per 100 grams of the respective fruit.

Fruit	Carbohydrate
Raisins	71 grams
Dehydrated prunes	67 grams
Dried apricots	55 grams
Bananas	18 grams
Grapes	17 grams
Figs	16 grams
Cherries	14 grams
Mangos	14 grams
Blueberries	12 grams
Pears	12 grams
Apples	11 grams
Kiwi	11 grams
Apricots	9 grams
Oranges	9 grams
Grapefruits	7 grams
Lemons	6 grams
Strawberries	5 grams
Blackberries	5 grams

Liquid Sugars:

In order to successfully get over your sugar addiction you'll need to say good-bye to all the liquid sugars that enter your body in the form of beverages, juices and others that have added sugar in them. Research has found that the body gives a distinct response when a person consumes a calorie-rich drink compared to a calorie-rich solid food; and the response isn't positive, in case you're wondering.

The bottom line is that liquid calories are less satisfying and people always want a little more of it. By avoiding drinks like colas, energy drinks, etc. and replacing them with vegetables, fruits and proteins you'll not only be able to break your sugar addiction but also save the body from a series of medical disasters like bone disease and cardiovascular injuries. Therefore, don't gulp down every drink that has "Natural" printed on it and be sure to take a look at the nutrition label.

Having said that, it is still important to drink lots of liquid products on a daily basis especially water, which is without a doubt extremely healthy even though it doesn't pack a lot of nutrients. The best thing to do to maintain water consumption is to carry a bottle of water with you every day, wherever you go. Tea & coffee are acceptable as well as long as you don't add spoonful of sugar into it! But watch out for cream as it contains sugar.

If you are one of those people who can't live without drinking sodas then think for a little while as to what you like about sodas? Most people just drink it for the fizz and carbonated water, and if that's the case with you then switch to "seltzer water". This product is not only carbonated and calorie free but also comes in a number of flavors. Mineral water is also great and some even come with added fizz. Still, if you can't go cold turkey on sodas then opt for diet ones as they contain lesser amount of sugar.

However, don't think of these sodas as you salvation as they still are harmful for your sugar addiction.

Another liquid drink that packs carbohydrates and is very much popular is milk that even though is natural, can be harmful for some people. Whether you're one of those who love to gulp down milk in the morning or eat it by adding it into a bowl of cereal, it is very likely that you always have a gallon of milk in your fridge.

This may come as a surprise to you but milk has sugar in it and I'm not even considering added one. The milk that you purchase from the supermarket or is delivered to your house contains a type of sugar known as lactose that is also found in other dairy products. You can counter this issue by switching to skimmed milk that has lesser fat content as well as reduced number of calories. In addition if you buy flavored milks that have chocolate or fruits then beware that they have a lot of added sugar to give the desired taste; it's best to stay away from them.

Cow's milk mostly consists of water and doesn't have a lot of sugar in it per se but lactose is a problem that can go a long way, especially for those who are lactose-intolerant. If you are lactose-intolerant then the best way to combat this is by drinking lactose-free milk as in the end milk is necessary for proper bone & body health. Once again, when purchasing these products, be sure to read the nutrition label and make sure that the milk doesn't pack any extra sugar.

If you are addicted to sugar and must drink milk to maintain your health then limit its consumption. Be one of those people who sip through a cup of coffee for hours, except use milk instead of coffee! Furthermore, avoid creamers, as they are high in sugar.

Hidden Sugars:

Hidden sugars are basically those sugars that surface in foods, often subtly, when you least expect them; examples of food items containing hidden sugars include sauces, dressings and condiments. As most of these products that pack hidden sugars are restricted when breaking your sugar addiction, you might want to take a look at the alternatives available to keep your foods tasty.

Spices are the best alternative when it comes to replacing sugar-containing products like salad dressings, ketchup and sauces. They are completely sugar free and add zeal & flavor to a food item. But avoid buying spices that have been processed as they may contain small amounts of carbohydrates. With the passage of time it is essential that you start making other changes as well like using limejuice instead of dressings in salad, or sprinkling thyme on top of chicken instead of barbecue sauce.

You can even create your very own marinade by putting a piece of meat or chicken in plastic bag and filling it up with your favorite spices and olive oil. Peanut butter also contains added sugar so try adding fresh nuts to a sandwich instead. And as the time passes you will notice that your taste & craving for sugar is dying and you no longer need to dip your tongue in honey to get satisfied. Once you stop consuming foods filled with sugar you're receptors will reset and their sensitivity will come back to normal

Maria Lexington

Conclusion

Thank you again for purchasing this book!

I hope this book was able to help you get rid of Small Intestinal Bacterial Growth. I did my best in trying to explain the possible solutions of this abnormality, which leads to several diseases that may turn chronic.

The next step is to apply this book practically in to your life and if it helps, recommend it to your friends and family!

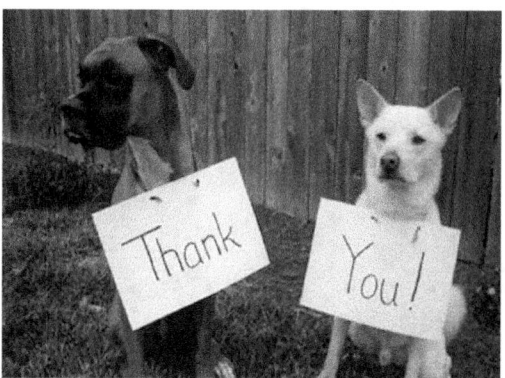

Finally, if you enjoyed this book, then I'd like to ask you for a favor, would you be kind enough to leave a review for this book on Amazon? It'd be greatly appreciated!

Thank you and good luck!